Dr. Donsbach tells you
what you always wanted to know about

Hypoglycemia
&
Diabetes

Kurt W. Donsbach, D.C., N.D., Ph.D.

©1994

Copyright © 1994

Printed in U.S.A.

From the Publisher:
This book does not intend to diagnose disease nor to provide specific medical advice. Its intention is solely to inform and to educate. The author and publisher intend that readers will use the information presented in this book in cooperation with a health professional.

INDEX

Index (continued)

HYPOGLYCEMIA

Hypoglycemia means low blood sugar. Although this condition was seldom heard of just a few years ago, today more and more physicians are finding that many of their patients who were real problems to diagnose are actually hypoglycemic. It only takes a minute to look at the myriad of symptoms to understand why this disorder can be masked and misdiagnosed.

SYMPTOMS OF HYPOGLYCEMIA

Headaches
Sudden Fatigue
Irritability
Insomnia
Forgetfulness
Anxiety
Depression
Crying Spells
Feeling of Faintness
Sudden Hunger
Exhaustion
Inability to Concentrate
Short Temper
Dizziness
Cold Sweats
Shakiness
Edema
Dry Mouth
Twitching of Eyelids
Uncontrollable Weight
  Gain

Overactivity in Children
Behavioral Problems
Seizures
Convulsions
Asthma
Hay Fever
Eczema
Hives
Sinusitis
Reduced Sex Drive
Stomach Pain
Clammy Skin
Digestive Disorders
Colitis
Diarrhea
Fearfulness
Blurred Vision
Shortness of Breath
Cold Extremities
Craving for Sweets,
  Alcohol, Coffee, or Cola

After reading that list of symptoms, one could say: "But that just about covers everybody." The unfortunate situation is that a tremendous number of people are hypoglycemic and never know it. They mask the symptoms by excessive eating of sweets, drinking alcohol, consuming large amounts of coffee, or smoking continually. Others are being treated for ulcers, gastritis, bad nerves, mental problems, heart disease, and any number of other misdiagnoses.

WHAT IS HYPOGLYCEMIA?

The condition of hypoglycemia is very complex when all the involved mechanisms in the body are detailed. For purposes of understanding, we shall use an overview to explain just what occurs.

The body's really not set up to handle the concentrated sugars which too often make up a large part of our diets. Although sugar is the fuel on which our entire body runs, the use of a concentrated form such as pastries, pies, sugar-coated cereals, or candy overloads the body's delicate control mechanism. The pancreas overreacts by producing too much insulin, depleting the blood sugar and causing the body to cry out for more food. Too often the wrong choice is made when this need is acute, and thus a vicious circle is established with side effects of malnutrition and all the attendant symptoms.

The malnutrition occurs because not enough protein-rich foods and vitamin and mineral containing vegetables are used. Instead, the convenience type foods take over a large percentage of the daily intake, and those are notorious for having nutrients processed out or even nonexistent to begin with. They are, in fact, often called "junk" foods.

CONVERSION MECHANISMS

Carbohydrates are converted to glucose in the gastrointestinal tract. The glucose is absorbed into the bloodstream, where it passes on to the liver. This marvelous organ then makes a decision as to the need for the sugar by the body. Some of the sugar that cannot be used as energy after it has been acted upon by insulin is converted to glycogen, an inert substance which is the instant reserve fuel for the body, and is stored in the liver and muscles (see figure 1). Glucose that cannot be stored as glycogen will be converted to fat. This can be one of the major causes of uncontrollable weight gain for certain individuals. (See figure 3.)

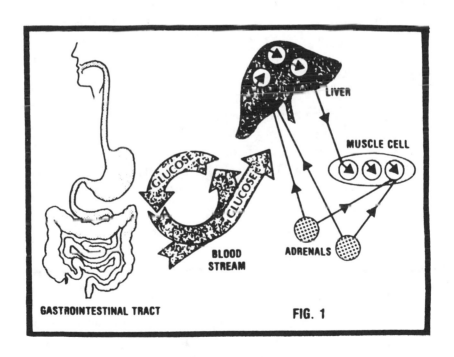

FIG. 1

In normal body function, there is a conversion mechanism which protects us against the rapid drop of blood sugar caused by the overproduction of insulin. The adrenal glands, which are the stress response glands, secrete a hormone which begins the process of changing glycogen back to glucose. This same response is brought into play when fear, anger, or emergency situations call for great strength. Such an expenditure of energy requires lots of fuel, so glycogen from the liver and muscles is immediately turned into glucose.

GLUCOSE AND GLYCOGEN CONVERSION

$$C_6H_{12}O_6 - H_2O \quad = \quad C_6H_{10}O_5$$

(Glucose)   (Glycogen)

$$C_6H_{10}O_5 + H_2O \quad = \quad C_6H_{12}O_6$$

(Glycogen)   (Glucose)

Glucose can be converted to an inert sugar (glycogen) by merely subtracting one molecule of water. It can also be reconverted in time of need (low blood sugar) back to glucose just by adding water back again. Glycogen is stored in the liver and muscle tissue.

Adrenalin, a hormone from the adrenals, assists in converting glycogen back to glucose.

FIGURE 2

If the glycogen conversion mechanism is not working well, the body has a backup mechanism. This consists of the conversion of amino acids and triglycerides into fuel. Amino acids are capable of converting to glucose but do so at the expense of tissue repair, manufacture of enzymes and hormones, and other essential processes that require amino acids. Since this provides emergency assistance only, you can easily imagine how the body suffers if it must take place on a continual basis.

Triglycerides (storage fat) are not converted readily to glucose but instead form ketone bodies which can be used in place of glucose as fuel. Since the body's need for amino acids is so critical, the triglycerides are the preferred source of substitute fuel.

The important thing to remember is that all these mechanisms are dependent upon hormones, and particularly upon adrenal hormones. Many physicians are convinced that the single most common cause of hypoglycemia is a poorly functioning adrenal system. Sluggish adrenals can cause slow conversion of glycogen to glucose in time of need, and if that occurs the craving for something sweet becomes overpowering.

GLUCOSE TO TRIGLYCERIDE CONVERSION

Formula For Glucose

$$C_6 H_{12} O_6$$

Formula For Triglycerides

$$C_{17} H_{35} O_8$$

Since only a relatively small amount of glucose is normally converted to glycogen, it is the next step that produces most fat in the body. This step converts glucose to triglycerides which are stored as fat in the body.

It can readily be seen that the major ingredients, carbon, hydrogen, and oxygen, are identical, only the amounts are different. This change takes place primarily in the liver although it may take place in the fat cell also.   **FIGURE 3**

HYPOGLYCEMIC SINCE BIRTH

Many infants are born with adrenal glands which function poorly because the mother had an adrenal problem. She may have had this problem for a long time, or may have been under considerable stress during pregnancy, or may have eaten a typical American diet high in refined carbohydrates and low in protein. The infant, in many cases, starts out in life with colic, diaper rash, respiratory disorders, and various adverse reactions to formulas. Formulas are too often given that are high in carbohydrates, which merely add to the innocent child's problems.

HYPOGLYCEMIC PROGRESSION

Assuming that most people are not born hypoglycemic, what causes some to become victims of this disorder and others to escape? The mechanism of hypoglycemia goes something like this:

1. Excessive intake of refined carbohydrates.
2. Rapid rise in blood sugar with resultant excess production of insulin by the pancreas.
3. Rapid decline in blood sugar because of the excess insulin, resulting in below normal blood sugar levels.
4. Adrenal response to convert glycogen to sugar for emergency.
5. Repetition of above pattern many times a day.
6. Tired adrenals don't respond as quickly.

7. Emergency! Body in danger of fainting, needs sugar fast!

8. Person eats or drinks a product with a high sugar content.

9. Blood sugar rises rapidly and cycle starts all over again.

Following such a progression, it is not difficult to see why hypoglycemics become physical and emotional yo-yos. When their blood sugar is elevated, they are feeling fine; when it drops, they have all kinds of symptoms.

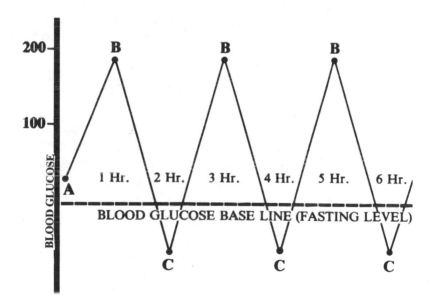

A. A food with a high concentration of sugar is consumed. Blood sugar begins to rise rapidly.

11

B. Because the intense sugar concentration of the food results in an abrupt rise in blood sugar, the pancreas is stimulated to produce the large amount of insulin which is needed to dispense the sugar. If the adrenals do not quickly produce a counterbalancing hormone to signal the end of insulin production, it is possible that blood sugar levels will fall below an acceptable level.

C. At this point, blood sugar levels are below normal and the signs of hypoglycemia are present: fatigue, headaches, irritability, etc. This will often be "remedied" by the consumption of either a concentrated sugar product or an adrenal stimulant such as coffee, cola or nicotine. The cycle is repeated over and over, all day long, unless measures are taken to restore normal function.

STRESS FACTORS

There are many kinds of stress in our environment, and all directly affect the adrenals, our stress glands. Some examples are infection, pain, overexertion, childbearing, burns, fractures, business problems, domestic disagreements, and drugs. Prolonged stress has a degrading effect on the body, particularly the adrenals, and eventually reduced efficiency to cope with stress ensues. Since the adrenals play such an important role in the hypoglycemic situation, such stress can bring on the condition or make it worse if it already exists. Hypoadrenocorticism, a condition characterized by low functioning of the adrenal glands, is very closely related to hypoglycemia.

Another factor which enters into this picture is the ability of an individual to whip his adrenal glands into functioning by the use of a variety of stimulant drugs. The two most common are coffee and tobacco. Both of these products are addictive because of their action on the adrenal glands. The stimulation of the adrenals energizes the glycogen conversion mechanism and the temporary rise in blood sugar gives the person a lift. It doesn't take much programming of the body for the individual to automatically reach for a cup of coffee or a cigarette when feeling down. In order to overcome his condition, the hypoglycemic must make up his mind to stop using both these drugs totally.

DIAGNOSIS

Although it is not used as perhaps it should be, the test for hypoglycemia is fairly simple. Approximately 100 grams of glucose (sugar) is administered after a fast of at least twelve hours. A blood sample is taken before the sugar is given and again each hour for a period of five to six hours. The deviations above and below the fasting level are diagnostic, particularly those below. Many individuals find that they feel faint and may even lose consciousness at the second or third hour because of the extreme drop in blood sugar levels.

It should be taken into consideration that the circumstances of this test are not those of everyday life. It is possible for the borderline hypoglycemic to show a fairly normal blood sugar curve in the laboratory, while under the stress of his job or other factors he may actually become hypoglycemic due to the added strain on his adrenal glands, which then respond sluggishly to the demand for glycogen conversion.

BLOOD SUGAR CURVES

Many ask what the glucose tolerance test tells the doctor. In a very simplified form, the following charts show some of the typical graphs that result from such a test. Although the degree of blood sugar drop is not always paralleled by the severity of the symptoms, it is a good indicator. Some individuals also react under stress conditions with a drastic drop in blood sugar levels, while under ordinary conditions their blood sugar levels are comparitively normal. This type of condition is the most difficult to diagnose. My suggestion to an individual who has hypoglycemia-type symptoms but has been told he or she is not hypoglycemic is to go on the hypoglycemic program. Nothing can be lost and the benefit can be immediate.

FOR THE FOLLOWING FOUR CHARTS

X   The fasting blood sugar level and the time when a measured amount of glucose is administered.

Y   Baseline blood sugar level. Any level below this is considered low blood sugar.

COMPARATIVELY NORMAL
BLOOD SUGAR CURVE

1. The six hour reading should be within five percent of the fasting level.
2. No point should fall below the baseline.
3. The one-hour level must rise at least fifty percent above the fasting level.

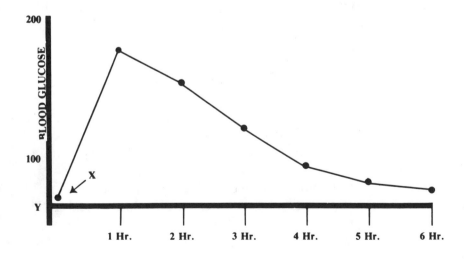

14

HYPOGLYCEMIC BLOOD SUGAR CURVE

This is only a relative comparison. There are severe cases where at the three-hour mark the blood sugar is already below the baseline. On the other hand, there are pre-hypoglycemics who dip one or two percent below the baseline at the fifth or sixth hour under test conditions, but under the daily stress of living may drop ten to twenty percent below the baseline with all the attendant emotional and physical symptoms. Thus the interpretations "borderline hypoglycemic" and "almost normal" are rather dangerous to the hypoglycemic patient because he may then consider his problems to be psychological and use tranquilizers, coffee, cigarettes, candy, or alcohol to cover up the symptoms.

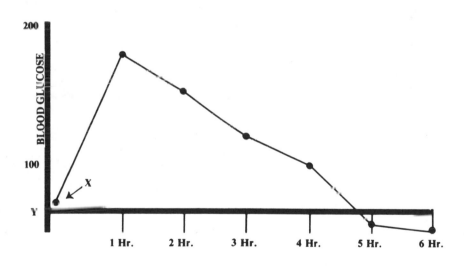

DIABETIC BLOOD SUGAR CURVE

Six hours after glucose intake, the blood sugar still has not returned to its high initial fasting level.

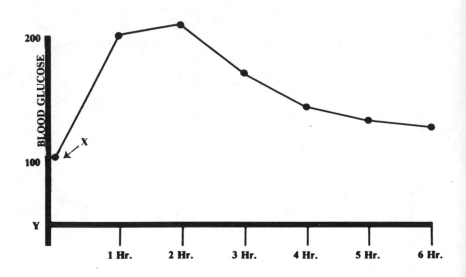

DIABETIC-HYPOGLYCEMIC
BLOOD SUGAR CURVE

A simple two or three hour glucose tolerance test on this individual would convince any physician that the patient is a diabetic. In reality, the patient is both diabetic and hypoglycemic at this point and a hypoglycemic diet will solve both problems, while an insulin program will create even more serious hypoglycemic symptoms. Also, the patient will have chronic difficulty regulating insulin intake. It is this type of patient that really points out the need for a full six-hour glucose tolerance evaluation.

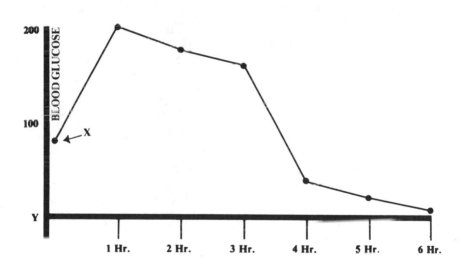

DON'T FORGET THE LIVER

We have been talking a great deal about the adrenal glands and their importance in dealing with the problems of hypoglycemia. Another organ in the body which plays a great part in blood sugar regulation is the liver, since it is in the liver that sugar is converted to glycogen for storage. The glycogen is stored in the liver and in muscle tissue, to be converted back to sugar again as needed. Thus it is easy to see the importance of healthy liver function for proper blood sugar levels.

The liver can be damaged or have its functional capacity reduced by several factors: excess alcohol consumption, tobacco, smog, infections, and toxic drugs. Fortunately, the liver regenerates faster than most organs, an indication of its importance to the body. Once the damaging factors are overcome, the liver will restore itself and carry out the many body functions it is designed to perform.

I highly recommend the Liver Cleansing Fast outlined later in this booklet for those who feel their liver could be a problem in their search for optimum health. The opinion exists in the minds of some that hypoglycemics are not supposed to go on fasts. I would like to point out one fact: in most cases the hypoglycemia is triggered by ingestion of a high carbohydrate food. In the Liver Cleansing Fast, no sugar is contained other than what might be naturally present in the lemon juice, and this will be so diluted that no emergency signal is sent to the pancreas for excess insulin. Thus, most hypoglycemics will reap nothing but benefits from the use of this fast.

HYPERINSULINISM

Hyperinsulinism is a term that some use almost synonymously with hypoglycemia. Literally interpreted, the word means an excess amount of insulin. We have seen how this excess occurs in the progression of hypoglycemia (pages 8 and 9). Another interesting tie-in of the adrenal glands and the pancreas is seen here. When the amount of insulin necessary to do the job on a given amount of sugar has been secreted, it is the job of an adrenal hormone to send a message to the pancreas to stop producing insulin. Sluggish adrenals will be late in this function, allowing overproduction of insulin with a resultant excessive lowering of the blood sugar.

DISASTROUS CONSEQUENCES

"I'm so tired all the time." "I don't seem to have any pep." "I can't stop feeling nervous." "I'm always depressed, even when things are okay." "I've tried every medication with no results." "I've been to every doctor around, and not one of them could find out what's wrong with me."

The above complaints are often heard, not only by doctors but by lay people as well. Hypoglycemia is a condition that frequently seems to evade the diagnostician because, until recently, it has not been seriously considered, even as a possiblity. In fact, many doctors would tell hypoglycemic patients to carry sugar lumps or candy at all times, to be taken whenever their symptoms arose. Unwittingly, these doctors were actually increasing the severity of their patients' disorder with this advice!

Various authorities have estimated that up to 100 million persons in the United States suffer from hypoglycemia. Such a high incidence of cases may be a significant factor contributing to our nation's difficulties, since hypoglycemics are not always functioning at their best and consequently can cause problems for themselves and for others. During the times when their blood sugar is low, hypoglycemics can become involved in needless arguments due to heightened irritability, their working efficiency can be drastically reduced, and they are susceptible to many severe mental and physical problems.

19

NUTRITIONAL SUPPLEMENTATION

It is this author's opinion that the control and reversal of hypoglycemia is directly related to furnishing the body with the nutrients that allow rebuilding, restoration, and rejuvenation of tissue cells to take place. Since the adrenals seem to be the organs most in need of supplementation, we can look at the specific nutrients which assist these glands.

Pantothenic Acid - For all practical purposes, one can say that this member of the B complex group of vitamins is in reality the catalyst for forming the adrenal hormones. In fact, one of the accepted signs of pantothenic acid deficiency is hypoadrena or low-functioning adrenals. It has been my experience that amounts of 1500 mg. or more are required on a daily basis.

Vitamin C - When this well-known vitamin is in low supply the adrenals have a tendency to become very congested with blood, to feel soft and mushy rather than firm to the touch, and even to develop internal hemorrhages. Obviously one cannot expect glands to operate at peak efficiency under these circumstances. The minimum amount that seems to be effective in overcoming a deficiency is 2,000 mg.

Potassium - Prolonged potassium deficiency results in hypertrophy (enlargement) of the adrenals and depletion of glycogen storage. The body's need for this essential mineral is two-and-a-half times as great as for calcium and phosphorous, which are the next most needed. Potassium requires chloride or it is readily excreted through the kidneys; therefore potassium chloride is the supplement of choice.

For an obscure and, in my opinion, unfounded reason, the Food and Drug Administration has seen fit to limit the amount of potassium choloride allowed in one tablet to 99 mg. This necessitates the use of multiple tablets to achieve the 900-1500 mg. which I have often found to be necessary for adequate daily supplementation.

GLANDULAR EXTRACTS

Locked within the nucleus of every cell in the body is coded genetic information used by the cell to rebuild itself when it begins to wear out. This cellular blueprint has been given the name deoxyribonucleic acid (DNA). When the cell does not receive adequte nutrients it has difficulty maintaining life, much less rebuilding anew. To stimulate the function of DNA, based on the concept that like cells help like cells, the use of glandular extracts has proven to be of value in assisting glands which have not been working up to par. Such glandular extracts, in this case adrenal, are available without prescription. I have found that a multiple glandular extract is far more efficient and effective than single glandular extracts.

RESTORATION PROGRAM

Now that we are familiar with hypoglycemia, its symptoms, causes and effects, it is time we thought about doing constructive restoration of the body. It is only with such a program that the relentless debilitation of the human body by a disorder such as hypoglyccmia can be overcome.

Many have said to me, "I don't know if I have hypoglycemia and I don't have the money for the tests and doctors." My answer is simple — try the program and if you feel better, stay on it! At the very worst, you will be following a good diet and your body will benefit from it.

TOTAL PROGRAM

Step One: Cleanse your body, particularly your liver, by going on the Liver Cleansing Fast outlined next. It can and has performed miracles for many—you are no exception. Over and above the obvious detoxification that occurs, mental clarity can be achieved beyond any other method.

Step Two: Follow the Carbohydrate Intolerant Diet Program very closely. On such a program you can expect to see changes in just days.

Step Three: Rebuild the glandular structure in your body, particularly the adrenals. We now know the DNA concentrates can have a tremendous rejuvenating effect on target glands.

Step Four: Because of the high carbohydrate diet which the hypoglycemic has been using, there are often some rather severe nutritional deficiencies present. The use of a very complete high-potency vitamin and mineral support is an absolute must for best and quickest results. Such a product, combined with an appropriate glandular extract, can be purchased without perscription. I offer a suggested guideline for choosing this supplement.

Step Five: Engage in a 3 times per week, 30 minute per time concentrated exercise program with your pulse rate up to at least 120 for the entire 30 minute period.

STRESS
PROTECTIVE NUTRIENTS

		% RDA
Vitamin A (Fish Liver Oil)	25,000 IU	500
Vitamin D (Fish Liver Oil)	1,000 IU	250
Vitamin E (d-Alpha Tocopheryl Acid Succinate)	400 IU	1333
Vitamin C (Ascorbic Acid)	2,000 mg	3332
Vitamin B-1 (Thiamine HCl)	50 mg	3332
Vitamin B-2 (Riboflavin)	50 mg	2940
Vitamin B-6 (Pyridoxine)	100 mg	5000
Vitamin B-12 (Cyanocobalamin)	500 mcg	8320
Niacinamide	50 mg	250
Pantothenic Acid (d-Calcium Pantothenate)	1,500 mg	15,000
Folic Acid	400 mcg	100
Biotin	100 mcg	33.3
Choline Bitartrate	100 mg	
Inositol	100 mg	
PABA (Para Amino Benzoic Acid)	50 mg	
Calcium (Dicalcium Phosphate & Oyster Shell)	500 mg	50
Magnesium (Oxide)	350 mg	62.5
Phosphorus (Dicalcium Phosphate)	100 mg	10
Potassium (Chloride)	400 mg	
Iron (Ferrous Fumerate)	15 mg	83
Zinc (Zinc Gluconate)	15 mg	100
Iodine (Kelp)	225 mcg	150
Copper (Copper Gluconate)	1 mg	50
Chromium (Chelated Chromium)	200 mcg	
Manganese (Manganese Gluconate)	20 mg	
RNA (Ribonucleic Acid)	10 mg	
Adrenal	100 mg	
Selenium (Chel. Selenium)	200 mcg	
Valerian	100 mg	

MULTI GLANDULARS
FEMALE

Adrenal	75 mg.
Ovarian	75 mg.
Thymus	75 mg.
Brain	75 mg.
Pituitary	15 mg.
Heart	75 mg.
Liver	75 mg.
Pancreas	75 mg.
Spleen	75 mg.
PABA	25 mg.
RNA	25 mg.
Choline	150 mg.
Pantothenic Acid	150 mg.

MALE

Adrenal	75 mg.
Brain	75 mg.
Heart	75 mg.
Kidney	75 mg.
Liver	75 mg.
Pancreas	75 mg.
Pituitary	15 mg.
Prostate	75 mg.
Spleen	75 mg.
Testes	75 mg.
Thymus	75 mg.
Zinc	25 mg.
PABA	25 mg.
RNA	25 mg.
Glycine	75 mg.
Glutamic Acid	75 mg.
Alanine	75 mg.

LIVER CLEANSING FAST

Materials Needed:

1. From 12 to 16 lemons daily depending on size. (If fresh lemons are unavailable, you can buy pure concentrated lemon juice.)
2. From 2 to 3 quarts of distilled water daily.
3. Small amount of honey.
4. One bottle of an herb combination containing garlic, quassia, black cohosh, chaparral, renugreek, red sage, and goldenseal.
5. One bottle of dietary fiber tablets. (May be called bran tablets.)

FIRST DAY: One and one-half cups freshly squeezed (or the equivalent of concentrate) lemon juice mixed with two quarts of distilled water and a little honey for palatability. This will be your total intake of fluid and food, so you may sip on it constantly. Take 2 of the herb tablets both morning and evening. Take 8 dietary fiber tablets in the morning and 8 in the afternoon, with a 10 ounce glass of the lemon mixture.

SECOND DAY: Repeat the mixing of approximately 2 ~ quarts of the lemon juice/distilled water/honey mixture and consume it during the day. Use 3 of the herb tablets morning and evening and 8 dietary fiber tablets twice daily.

THIRD DAY: Repeat the mixing of the approximately 21/2 quarts of the lemon juice/distilled water/honey mixture and consume it during the day. Use 4 of the herb tablets morning and evening and 8 dietary fiber tablets twice daily.

This is the end of the concentrated detoxifying, but the first week after the program is extremely important, regarding its lasting benefits. The following suggestions as to eating should be observed:

FOURTH AND FIFTH DAY: Stop using the lemon juice/distilled water/honey mixture, but continue the use of 2 herb tablets morning and evening. Also, use 8 dietary fiber tablets morning and afternoon. Drink all you wish of tomato juice, carrot juice, grape juice (dilute the grape juice with about one-third spring water) and other vegetable or fruit juices. Do not use citrus juices. Consume all the fresh spring water you wish.

SIXTH AND SEVENTH DAY: Add raw fruits and vegetables to your regimen, maintaining herb and dietary fiber tablet intake as before. Consume all the fresh juices that you wish.

EIGHTH DAY: Add yogurt and/or cottage cheese. Continue dietary fiber and herb tablets twice during the day.

NINTH DAY: Add lightly steamed vegetables to allowed foods. Reduce dietary fiber tablet intake to 12. Continue taking 4 herb tablets on a daily basis.

TENTH DAY: If desired, add a small portion of meat to one meal. Seeds, nuts, or eggs are just as acceptable. Reduce dietary fiber tablets to 4 in the morning and 4 in the afternoon. Use 4 herb tablets as before.

ELEVENTH DAY FORWARD: Follow the Creative Restoration Diet. Adjust dietary fiber tablets according to personal need; lower bowel gas and foul odored stools are indications of increased need for dietary fiber. You may now discontinue the herb tablets.

DIET PROGRAM FOR
CARBOHYDRATE INTOLERANTS

Early Mini-Meal . . . . Choice of allowed fruit.
(Upon Rising)

Breakfast . . . . Six ounces of tomato juice, one or two eggs with choice of meat, cheese or cottage cheese. ONLY ONE slice (toasted and buttered if desired) of whole grain bread (not essential). No cold cereals allowed.

Mid-Morning Mini-Meal . . . . . Eight ounces of a multiple source protein drink.*

Lunch . . . . Meat, fish, eggs, or cheese; vegetables as desired, permissable salads beverage.

Mid-Afternoon Mini-Meal . . . Eight ounces of multiple source protein drink OR fresh fruit or vegetable juice.

**Pre-Dinner Appetite
Stabilizer** . . . . Six ounces vegetable juice.

Dinner . . . . Soup if desired (not thickened with flour), vegetables, portion of meat, fish, or poultry; one slice of whole grain bread with plenty of butter if desired, beverage.

Bedtime Mini-Meal . . . . Six to eight ounces of multiple source protein drink.

NOTE: At least ⅔ of the daily intake should be consumed before mid-afternoon. It is not wise to eat a large dinner.

NOTE: Some form of daily exercise is highly recommended, e.g., bicycle riding, badminton, tennis, jogging, isometric, weight lifting, square dancing, calisthenics, etc.

THIS DIET WILL BE AS SUCCESSFUL AS YOU ARE FAITHFUL IN FOLLOWING IT.

* Your doctor will recommend the protein concentrate for you that will be used for your protein drink. Tomato or V-8 juice is an excellent base liquid for this health builder.

SELECTION CHART

CHOICE GROUP

MEATS - Veal, beef, lamb, fish, poultry are the best choices. Ham, bacon, sausage and other processed meats should be eliminated.

FRUITS - Apricots, apples, berries, melons, peaches, pears, pineapple, tangerines, grapefruit, oranges, cantloupes, strawberries, watermelons, plums.

JUICES - Any unsweetened fruit or vegetable juices, except grape or prune juice. *Warning:* fruit juices may be too concentrated for some, dilute with water.

VEGETABLES - Any vegetable except those listed below.

BEVERAGES - Herb tea, cereal coffee substitute. No sugar added.

DESSERTS - Fruits, preferably eaten 3 hours after meal.

NOTE: Fruits should be raw or cooked without sugar. If you use canned fruits, be sure they are packed in water. Raw fruits are best.

AVOID GROUP

MEATS - Ham, bacon, sausage, and other processed meats.

JUICES - Grape juice and prune juice.

VEGETABLES - Hominy, yams, potatoes (except raw or baked, twice weekly), corn, dried beans.

BEVERAGES - All alcoholic beverages, all soft drinks, coffee, tea.

PREPARED FOODS - White flour bakery products, spaghetti, macaroni, noodles, gravies.

DESSERTS — Candies and other sugar sweets, such as cakes, pies, pastries, custard, jello, ice cream, sherbets, puddings.

CLASSIFICATION OF FOODS
(According to Carbohydrate Content)

VEGETABLES

3 Percent	6 Percent	15 Percent	20 Percent	25 Percent
Asparagus	Beans, String	Artichokes	Beans, Dried	Rice, boiled
Bean Sprouts	Beets	Beans, Kidney	Beans, Lima	Potato, Sweet
Beet Greens	Brussel sprouts	Hominy	Corn	Yams
Broccoli	Carrots	Oyster plant	Potato, White	
Cabbage	Chives	Parsnips		
Cauliflower	Collards	Peas, Green		
Celery	Dandelion Greens			
Chard, Swiss	Eggplant			
Cucumber	Kale			
Endive	Kohirabie			
Lettuce	Leeks			
Mushrooms	Okra			
Mustard Greens	Onions			
Radishes	Parsley			
Sauerkraut	Peppers, Red			
Spinach	Pimento			
Squash	Pumpkins			
Tomatoes	Rutabagas			
Tomato Juice	Turnips			
Watercress				

FRUITS

3 Percent	6 Percent	15 Percent	20 Percent	25 Percent
Cantaloupe	Apricots	Apples	Bananas	
Rhubarb	Blackberries	Blueberries	Figs	
Strawberries	Cranberries	Cherries	Prunes	
Watermelon	Currants	Grapes		
	Gooseberries	Kumquats		
	Grapefruit	Loganberries		
	Guava	Mangoes		
	Melons	Mulberries		
	Lemons	Pears		
	Limes	Pineapple		
	Oranges	Pomegranates		
	Papayas			
	Peaches			
	Plums			
	Raspberries			
	Tangerines			

In making your choice of vegetables, you may use all the 3% and 6% selections you wish every day. Twice weekly, choose one from the 15%, 20%, or 25% group as a change.

In making your choice of fruits, it is desirable that you limit the amount to one 3% selection during the first days of your diet. As you progress, other choices can be made.

And so you have a program to nutritionally support your body, helping restore biochemical balance which can lead to some very noticible changes in function.

Let me just give a few nutrients which have special functions in controlling hypoglycemia:

Cysteine: An amino acid which may have an effect on excess insulin by reducing one or more of this chemicals disulfide bonds thus altering its shape and function. The most common and most concentrated source of cysteine is the egg containing approximately 250 mg of cysteine per large egg.

Vitamin C: A must when cysteine is used because it prevents the oxidation of cysteine to cystine which may be a factor in kidney stone formation. Use at least 3 times the amount of vitamin C as cysteine.

Let me give you some things to consider regarding insulin which, as we have discussed, is often overproduced in hypoglycemia.

Evidence supports the idea that insulin can promote deletrious changes in the cardiovascular system. It is well known that most insulin-using diabetics eventually develop cardiovascular complications such as atherosclerosis. Some scientists now think it is insulin that is primarily responsible for these changes. Insulin can cause lipids to be deposited in arterial walls. It also increases fat storage in adipose (fatty) tissues by stimulating the synthesis of lipids and inhibiting their breakdown.

Some sugars that are more complex in structure than sucrose (table sugar) do not cause insulin release and, therefore, do not have the side effects mentioned in the previous paragraph. These noninsulin-requiring sugars include sorbitol, mannitol, inositol (muscle sugar, a B vitamin), and xylitol. Fructose releases less insulin over a longer time and consequently causes fewer problems than sucrose (cane or beet sugar) or glucose. There is evidence, however, that fructose elevates triglycerides more than sucrose does. Honey and brown sugar have the same type of insulin-releasing effect as sucrose and therefore offer no advantages in this respect. Insulin suppresses growth hormone release and may, therefore, impair the immune system's ability to destroy atherosclerotic plaques, bacteria, viruses, and cancer cells. Since an important amount of growth hormone is released during the first hour and a half of sleep, it is particularly important not to eat table sugar or foods containing large quantities of it within a few hours of bedtime.

For many cases of adult-onset-type diabetes, the best medicine is control of body weight. If you keep yourself slender, you will probably require little or possible no insulin shots—and you will be in less danger of developing cardiovascular disease and blindness. You should not try rapid weight reduction by fasting if you are a diabetic, and you should, of course remain under your doctor's close care.

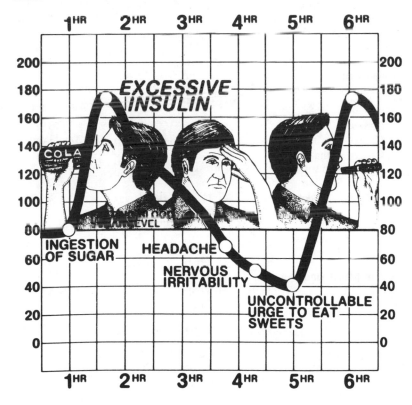

HIDDEN SUGARS IN FOODS

Food Item	Size of Portion	Approximate sugar content in teaspoonfuls of granulated sugar
CANDIES		
Average Chocolate Milk Bar (ex: Hershey bar)	1 (1½ oz.)	2½
Chewing Gum	1 stick	½
Chocolate Cream	1 piece	2
Butterscotch Chew	1 piece	1
Chocolate Mints	1 piece	2
Fudge	1 oz. square	4½
Gum Drop	1	2
Hard Candy	4 oz.	20
Lifesavers	1	⅓
Peanut Brittle	1 oz.	3½
CANNED FRUIT & JUICES		
Canned Apricots	4 halves & 1 Tbsp. syrup	3½
Canned Fruit Juices (sweetened)	½ Cup	2
Canned Peaches	2 halves & 1 Tbsp. syrup	3½
Fruit Salad	½ Cup	3½
Fruit Syrup	2 Tbsp.	2½
Stewed Fruits	½ Cup	2
DAIRY PRODUCTS		
Ice Cream	⅓ pt. (3½ oz.)	3½
Ice Cream Bar	1 (depending on size)	1-7
Ice Cream Cone	1	3½
Ice Cream Soda	1	5
Ice Cream Sundae	1	7
Malted Milk Shake	1 (10 oz. glass)	5
JAMS & JELLIES		
Apple Butter	1 Tbsp.	1
Jelly	1 Tbsp.	4-6
Orange Marmalade	1 Tbsp.	4-6
Peach Butter	1 Tbsp.	1
Strawberry Jam	1 Tbsp.	4
DESSERTS, MISCELLANEOUS		
Apple Cobbler	½ Cup	3
Blueberry Cobbler	½ Cup	3
Custard	½ Cup	2
French Pastry	1 (4 oz. piece)	5
Jello	1 Cup	4½

Food Item	Size of Portion	Approximate sugar content in teaspoonfuls of granulated sugar

BEVERAGES

Cola Drinks	1 (6 oz. bottle or glass)	3½
Cordials	1 (¾ oz. glass)	1½
Ginger Ale	6 oz.	5
Hi-Ball	1 (6 oz. glass)	2½
Orange-Ade	1 (8 oz. glass)	5
Root Beer	1 (10 oz. bottle)	4½
Seven-Up	1 (6 oz. bottle or glass)	3¾
Soda Pop	1 (8 oz. bottle)	5
Sweet Cider	1 cup	6
Whiskey Sour	1 (3 oz. glass)	1½

CAKES & COOKIES

Angel Food	1 (4 oz. piece)	7
Apple Sauce Cake	1 (4 oz. piece)	5½
Banana Cake	1 (2 oz. piece)	2
Cheese Cake	1 (4 oz. piece)	2
Chocolate Cake (Plain)	1 (4 oz. piece)	6
Chocolate Cake (Iced)	1 (4 oz. piece)	10
Coffee Cake	1 (4 oz. piece)	4½
Cup Cake (Iced)	1	6
Fruit Cake	1 (4 oz. piece)	5
Jelly-Roll	1 (2 oz. piece)	2½
Orange Cake	1 (4 oz. piece)	4
Pound Cake	1 (4 oz. piece)	5
Sponge Cake	1 (1 oz. piece)	2
Strawberry Shortcake	1 serving	4
Brownies (unfrosted)	1 (¾ oz.)	3
Chocolate Cookies	1	1½
Fig Newtons	1	5
Ginger Snaps	1	3
Macaroons	1	6
Nut Cookies	1	1½
Oatmeal Cookies	1	2
Sugar Cookies	1	1½
Chocolate Eclair	1	7
Cream Puff	1	2
Donut (Plain)	1	3
Donut (Glazed)	1	6
Snail	1 (4 oz. piece)	4½

DIABETES

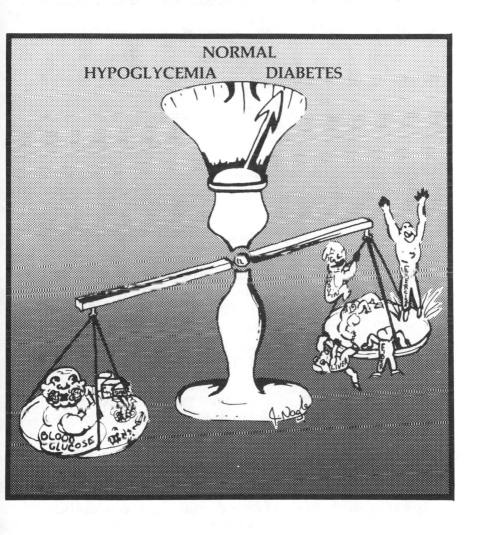

DIABETES

Although there are other forms of diabetes than diabetes mellitus, it is by far the most common and the basic subject of this booklet. Even though there are records of diabetes more than 2300 years ago, it still persists as one of the most difficult diseases to treat. Insulin, once thought to be the saviour of the diabetic, now is known to only be an adjunct to its symptomatic management and 50% or more of the diabetic population have severe difficulty in regulating dosages of this hormone.

Let's examine just what diabetes really is. By definition diabetes is a nutritional disease since it is involved with the body's ability or lack of ability to properly metabolize food consumed. The common belief that it is due to a lack of proper function of the beta cells of the pancreas has been found seriously wanting. Hyperfunction of the adrenal or pituitary glands can produce it, as can malfunction of the liver or the alpha cells of the pancreas.

What really becomes evident is the complexity of diabetes and the fact that the body finds itself unable to adequately utilize sugar (properly called glucose).

SYMPTOMS

The symptoms of diabetes often are subtle in the beginning stages, but here are some very excellent questions which might lead one to have a test for diabetes.

In the past two months have you:

1. Been unusually thirsty?
2. Been passing more urine than normal?
3. Noticed that small wounds heal slowly?
4. Been unusually tired?
5. Had others tell you that your breath smelled acid?
6. Been more prone to infections than usual?
7. Lost weight other than a restriction of food?
8. Had an unexplained loss of sexual desire?

If your answer to one or more of these questions is yes, you may wish to have a blood test for excess sugar.

There are simple home tests that can be performed as a screening mechanism and, in my opinion, are something that everyone should do every six months. These tests use a reagent, usually in the form of a strip of paper which is dipped in a sample of the urine or the urine may be voided directly on the strip.

PROCEDURE

To my knowledge, there are three paper or plastic strip tests for glucose in the urine:

1. Clinistix (Ames)
2. Tes-Tape (Lilly)
3. Diastix (Ames)

All are very accurate, but in order to insure such accuracy, it is necessary to follow the simple time instructions which come with the test. All these tests are readily available at your local pharmacy.

I should also caution you that you should discontinue taking vitamin C for 24 hours before the test, or if you are taking the drugs L-Dopa or Methyl Dopa, inaccurate results may occur. You must understand that neither vitamin C or the drugs mentioned produce diabetes. They merely cause a false reading due to chemical reactions when they come in contact with the chemicals on the reagent strip.

The test strips all contain a chemical which reacts to glucose. Increasing concentrations create color changes in the strip which can be matched with a control color panel on the container to give an approximation of the amount of sugar in the urine.

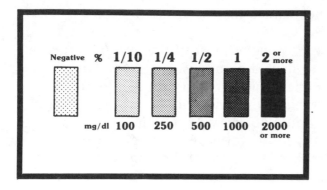

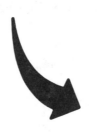

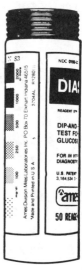

During my investigation of this metabolic condition we call diabetes, I was impressed with the mountain of information available but was distressed that so little actually has been accomplished to decrease the incidence. Part of the problem lies in the complexities which face anyone who begins to really research diabetes. Is it primarily hereditary? Is it due to a malfunctioning of the beta cells of the pancreas? Is it really due to a pituitary aberration? Since over 50% of the adult onset diabetics have adequate or more than adequate insulin, is it due to an excess of glucagon, which is an insulin antagonist? Is it because the individual just ate too much sugar? Does obesity lead to diabetes? Is a virus involved?

I could go on and on with the possibilities, but the purpose of this booklet will be to give you my best conclusions after carefully examining as much information as is available. Routine testing with a urine glucose reagent strip can be your best control, since you will discover your tendency toward diabetes this way very early, thus making it easier to control.

WHAT IS INSULIN?

In order to understand diabetes, the most frequently related word is insulin. This hormone, produced by the pancreas, has a very important function. Many think that it "burns up" glucose in the blood stream. It does not! The easiest description I have for insulin is that of a door-man at a very elegant hotel, who wishes to show you the way to your destination. Insulin acts to "open the door" of the cell so glucose may enter. If the glucose is ushered into a muscle cell, it may be combined with oxygen to create energy with the waste products of carbon dioxide and water remaining, or if it enters a muscle cell that is not in need of energy at that time, the glucose may be converted to glycogen, which is an inert storage form of glucose capable of being changed back to glucose when energy is needed.

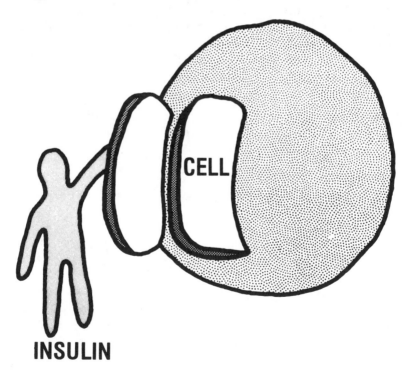

CELL

INSULIN

GLUCOSE

MUSCLE CELL

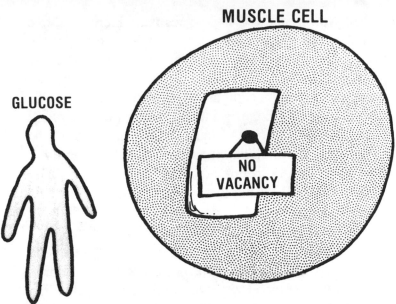

If no energy is needed and if the glycogen warehouses are full, the glucose will end up in a fat cell where it is converted to triglycerides, the storage fat which the body accumulates in times of plenty. Under certain circumstances this can happen right in the liver (the conversion of glucose to trigylcerides) and the resulting fats are poured into the blood stream, often creating a "sludging" effect which can create oxygen problems.

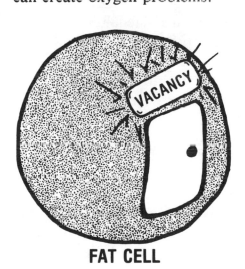

FAT CELL

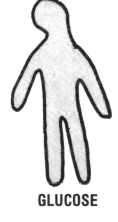

GLUCOSE

But, you might ask, if diabetes is an increase above normal in the glucose level and if 50% or more of the diabetics have normal insulin, what is happening? Good question! The most accepted answer is that the insulin receptors (you might compare them with door knobs on a door) become insulin resistant and the hormone just can't get its job done. Glucose begins to pile up in the blood, the body tries to dump it via the urine so you begin to drink more water in a desperate effort to flush the potentially dangerous ingredient out through the kidneys.

Our body needs the glucose, since this is the fuel that we use, just like a car that has a gas tank full of fuel but a carburetor that won't allow the gas to reach the combustion chamber. At this time I should make it clear that there ARE diabetics who respond very well to injected insulin. The mechanism is quite simple; these may be the percentage of diabetics who really have a pancreas problem and are not producing enough insulin, or the extra insulin in some way overwhelms the resistance to insulin just by volume and glucose gets into the cell.

I really want to state one of the most accepted facts about diabetes: "Almost All Adult Onset Diabetes Can Be Controlled Totally By Dietary Changes." The only problem with this common knowledge is that it requires some rather heavy commitment on the part of both the doctor and the patient. The doctor must take the time to educate the patient about his body and how it uses food, the patient must often drastically change food habits. Neither is easy, and often the lackadaisical attitude on the part of both ends up with disastrous results for the patient.

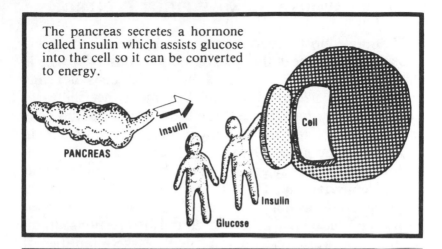

The pancreas secretes a hormone called insulin which assists glucose into the cell so it can be converted to energy.

PANCREAS

Insulin

Cell

Insulin

Glucose

Glucose can be converted to an inert sugar (glycogen) by merely subtracting one molecule of water. It can also be reconverted in time of need (low blood sugar) back to glucose just by adding water back again. Glycogen is stored in the liver and muscle tissue.

$$C_6H_{12}O_6 - H_2O = C_6H_{10}O_5$$
(Glucose)   (Glycogen)

$$C_6H_{10}O_5 + H_2O = C_6H_{12}O_6$$
(Glycogen)   (Glucose)

Adrenalin, a hormone from the adrenals, assists in converting glycogen back to glucose.

Since only a relatively small amount of glucose is normally converted to glycogen, it is the next step that produces most fat in the body. This step converts glucose to triglycerides which are stored as fat in the body.

Formula for Glucose $C_6H_{12}O_6$
Formula for Triglycerides $C_{17}H_{35}O_6$

It can readily be seen that the major ingredients, carbon, hydrogen, and oxygen, are identical, only the amounts are different. This change takes place primarily in the liver although it may take place in the fat cell also.

43

THE IMPORTANCE OF WEIGHT CONTROL

The single most important reason why weight control is of such importance in the control of adult-onset diabetes is that the responsiveness to insulin of fat cells depends largely on the size of the fat cell. In man, once the early days of infancy have passed, the total amount of fat cells in the body is fixed and no longer increase in numbers in response to the needs of additional fat storage. As an individual progressively gains weight, the individual fat cells enlarge considerably. The larger adipose cells are, the less responsive to insulin they are. Thus, adipose cells of overweight individuals shows a diminished response to insulin and, in fact, require abnormally large quantities of insulin to sustain normal carbohydrate metabolism and tolerance.

You will remember our little schematic that followed glucose to the muscle cell, then to the fat cell. If neither is willing to accept, that glucose is trapped in the blood stream. Weight loss with a reduction in size of the fat cell, allows normal sensitivity to insulin and the carbohydrate metabolism once again comes into balance. This brings up the question: What is the proper weight for me?

WHAT IS THE "RIGHT" WEIGHT FOR YOU?

Stunning new medical evidence shows you're not really overweight if you're only 15 to 20 percent heavier than your "ideal" weight. That's because those height-weight tables distributed by Metropolitan Life Insurance Co. — and widely used by doctors — are all wrong, experts have discovered in a series of studies. In fact, say the experts, you'll actually live longer if you're quite a bit heavier than your so-called perfect weight as shown on the famous tables.

"There's something about being moderately overweight that's good for you," said Dr. Reubin Andres, clinical director of the prestigious National Institute of Aging.

Dr. Andres did an exhaustive review of 17 longterm

health studies—and came up with these "shocking" findings:

"Several of the studies show that people who were at or slightly below their ideal weight (as shown on the Metropolitan tables) have a higher mortality rate at every age than those who were moderately overweight.

"None of the studies show shortened life expectancy for persons who are up to 20 percent overweight. Some show no shortened life expectancy for those up to 30 percent overweight!"

Dr. Andres cautioned that obesity is "devastating" for people with serious medical problems such as diabetes, high blood pressure and a high cholesterol level. But if you don't have such problems, there's no reason to worry about being slightly overweight, he declared.

A Harvard University researcher, Dr. Carl C. Seltzer, Ph.D., concluded that the data on which the Metropolitan tables are based — published by the Society of Actuaries in 1959 — is completely off-base.

"The insurance companies claim that your mortality rate increases proportionately to how much overweight you are.

"I analyzed the Society of Actuaries own figures and showed that this isn't true," said Dr. Seltzer, an honorary research associate.

"Doctors and insurance companies have been following these guidelines put out by Metropolitan and this has needlessly instilled fear into millions of Americans — causing them to worry needlessly about being overweight when they really aren't.

"Unless you are grossly overweight, there is no more than an average risk."

Renowned nutritionist and author Dr. Neil Solomon — formerly assistant professor of psychiatry at Johns Hopkins medical School — flatly stated:

"The Metropolitan height-weight tables are a lot of bunk! I have found that being overweight by about 15 percent, using the tables as your guideline, will actually help you live longer.

45

"That's a startling statistic — and it should put at ease millions of Americans who thought they were too fat."

Other experts agree that Metropolitan's tables are totally unrealistic.

"If most people got right down to the Metropolitan's figures they would actually be underweight, unhealthy and more susceptible to illness and disease," said Dr. Frank W. Barr, diplomate of the American Board of Bariatric Medicine.

Typical of the studies analyzed by Dr. Andres was a 14 year Northwestern University survey of 1,233 people.

In that project, researchers found people with the lowest mortality were 25 to 35 percent overweight, said Dr. Alan R. Dyer, Ph.D., Associate professor of community health and preventive medicine, who co-authored the study with Dr. Howard A. Lindberg and two other experts.

Another study was the famous Framingham Heart Study sponsored by the National Heart, Lung, and Blood Institute.

This showed that the lowest death rates were among men and women aged 40 to 59 whose average weight was 15 to 20 percent over their ideal weight shown on the Metropolitan tables.

The Society of Actuaries is just completing a new study — and will publish a report listing ideal weights that are at least 10 pounds higher than those now shown on the Metropolitian tables.

Metropolitan and other top life insurance companies say they plan to revise their charts upward accordingly.

But even after the chart weights are increased, they'll still be too low, according to experts.

The following charts are a rational attempt to bring scientific facts into the arena of weight guidelines. In order to determine if you are small, medium or large boned, measure your wrist with a common tape measure and use the following parameters:

Men: 6 inches - small boned
7 inches - medium boned
8 inches - large boned

MEN (ages 25 and over)

Weight in Pounds According to Frame (With Indoor Clothing)

HEIGHT (with shoes on, 1-inch heels)		SMALL FRAME	MEDIUM FRAME	LARGE FRAME
Feet	Inches			
5	2	129-139	137-150	146-164
5	3	133-143	140-155	150-168
5	4	137-146	144-158	153-173
5	5	140-150	147-162	157-177
5	6	144-155	151-167	161-182
5	7	149-159	156-171	165-188
5	8	153-164	161-177	171-194
5	9	158-169	165-182	176-199
5	10	163-175	170-187	181-204
5	11	168-180	175-193	186-210
6	0	173-185	180-199	192-216
6	1	177-189	185-205	197-222
6	2	185-195	189-211	203-228
6	3	187-200	195-217	209-234
6	4	192-205	201-223	213-240

Women: 5½ inches - small boned
6 inches - medium boned
6½ inches - large boned

WOMEN (ages 25 and over)

Weight in pounds According to Frame (With Clothing)

HEIGHT (with shoes on, 2-inch heels)		SMALL FRAME	MEDIUM FRAME	LARGE FRAME
Feet	Inches			
4	10	106-114	111-124	121-139
4	11	109-117	114-128	123-142
5	0	111-121	117-132	127-146
5	1	115-124	121-135	130-150
5	2	118-128	125-139	134-153
5	3	122-132	128-142	138-157
5	4	126-135	132-147	141-162
5	5	129-139	135-152	146-166
5	6	133-144	140-158	151-171
5	7	138-148	145-163	156-176
5	8	142-153	150-168	160-181
5	9	147-158	154-172	165-174
5	10	152-164	159-177	170-192
5	11	157-169	164-182	175-198
6	0	162-174	169-187	180-204

(For girls between 18 and 25, subtract 1 pound
for each year under 25)

In adult-onset diabetes, weight reduction to the mid-levels of the foregoing chart is the only therapy that many need to control symptoms and live a normal life.

TOTAL ELIMINATION OF
REFINED CARBOHYDRATES

A well established characteristic of the diabetic is an elevated cholesterol and triglyceride level. Low-density lipoprotein (LDL) levels are almost always elevated, whereas high-density lipoprotein (HDL) levels are usually lower than normal. LDL's and HDL's are part of the cholesterol complex. There is evidence that these two cholesterol fractions and their ratio one to another is a better index of impending heart disease than any other. You might ask, "Well, since these are fats, shouldn't I cut all the fats in my diet?"

The answer is not that simple. Numerous research studies have indicated that the very best way to reduce the levels of LDL's and increase the levels of HDL's is to totally eliminate refined carbohydrates from the diet.

Also, the triglyceride levels are increased in proportion to the amount of refined, concentrated sucrose in the diet. Certain statements have been made that this elevation of triglycerides is in direct relation to the glucose in the diet, but evidence I have makes this seem quite erroneous.

Consider this research by Milton Winitz, J. Graff, and D.A. Seeman, printed in the *Archives of Biochemistry and Biophysics 108,* 576 (1964), and M. Winitz et al., in the *American Journal of Clinical Nutrition 23,* 525, 546 (1970). These investigators studied 18 subjects, who were kept in a locked institution, without access to other food, during the whole period of the study (about six months). After a preliminary period with ordinary food, they were placed on a chemically well-defined small-molecule diet (17 amino acids, a little fat, vitamins, essential minerals, and glucose as the only carbohydrate.) The only significant physiological change that was found was in the concentration of cholesterol in the blood serum which decreased rapidly for each of the 18 subjects.

The average concentration in the initial period, on ordinary food, was 227 milligrams per deciliter. After two weeks on the glucose diet it had dropped to 173, and after another two weeks to 160. The diet was then changed by replacing one quarter of the glucose with sucrose, with all of the other dietary constituents kept the same. Within one week the average cholesterol concentration had risen from 160 to 179, and after two more weeks to 208. The sucrose was then replaced by glucose. Within one week the average cholesterol concentration had dropped to 175, and it continued dropping, leveling off at 150 - 77 less than the initial value.

This important experiment, in which the only change made was to replace some of the glucose in the diet with sucrose and then return to the sucrose-free diet, shows conclusively that an increased intake of sucrose leads to an increased level of blood cholesterol. Levels of triglycerides are even more sensitive to the concentration of the sucrose than is the cholesterol level. The sucrose-cholesterol triglyceride effect is understandable, because it is known that fructose, formed in the digestion of sucrose, undergoes reactions in the body which lead to the formation of these two blood fats. So, although fructose may not provoke an insulin response, it can so sludge up your blood with fats that important functions are inhibited.

It is my opinion that the most logical reason for this phenomena could follow this pattern:
1. Excess sucrose intake leads to
2. High levels of fructose which is converted into
3. Triglycerides which may lodge on the exterior of the fat cells which interfere with
4. Insulin receptor sites, closing the door to glucose
5. Which raises the blood sugar and produces
6. Diabetes

The above is predicated upon the fact that as many as 9 out of 10 adult onset diabetics have more than normal circulating insulin and are not insulin dependent.

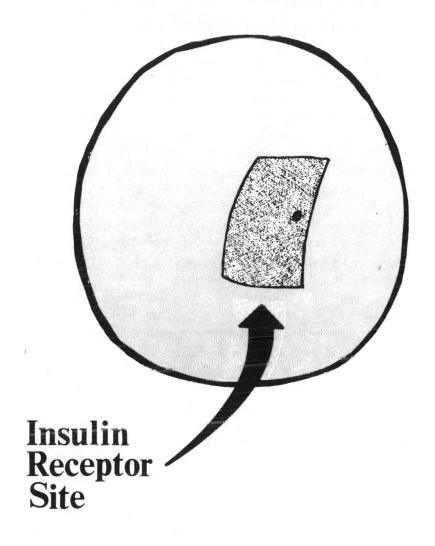

Insulin Receptor Site

The insulin receptor site might be likened to the doorknob on a door. There are several such receptors on each normal cell, but as a fat cell gets larger the number of sites decrease, conversely, as one loses weight, the reverse occurs. One research paper indicated that a reduction in weight by 10 percent increased the insulin receptor site availability by a factor of ten.

GLUCOSE TOLERANCE FACTOR

Recent attention has focused upon a little known mineral which lies at the center of a molecular structure which facilitates the transfer of glucose into the cell. Although total mechanisms are not fully understood, GTF (Glucose Tolerance Factor) appears to be a mediator between the insulin and the insulin receptors on the cell. It is made up of the mineral chromium, two glutamic acids and three niacins. Primary grown yeast is the best source of GTF, about two tablespoons a day seem to be adequate. Many report excellent results with the mineral chromium all by itself. Some very surprising response has been demonstrated with the use of either the yeast compound or the mineral - chromium.

It has been so effective for some who were taking insulin, that they wound up in the hospital with acute hypoglycemia, when they took a dosage of four or more tablespoons of yeast! This only proves that the diabetes in that individual was not due to a lack of insulin but due to a lack of insulin receptor sites in good working order. It is good common sense, if you are taking insulin, that you institute corrective measures which might be suggested in this booklet with caution. Know the signs of an overdosage of insulin - nervousness, trembling, rapid breathing, damp sweaty skin, and finally unconsciousness. The immediate treatment for this is some form of readily available sugar - particularly if the patient loses consciousness. Ordinary table sugar under the tongue works well in an emergency. (It is better than orange juice for example, because the fluid could enter the lung and create more problems.) When changing your diet radically or instituting any other change in life style, the insulin taking diabetic should always be alert for signs of body changes, and possibly adjust their insulin intake accordingly.

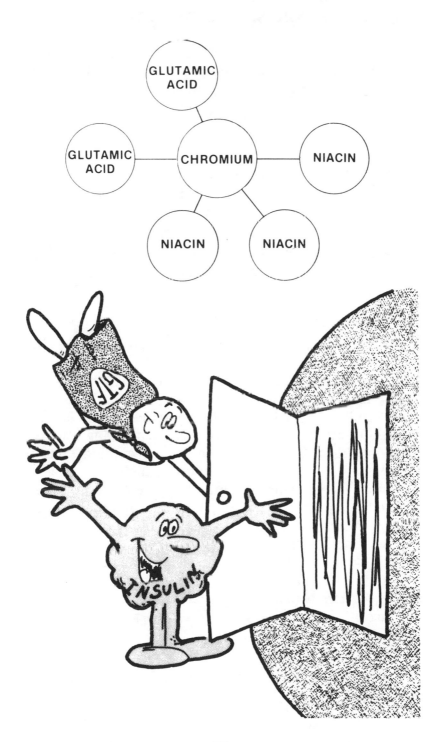

53

EXERCISE AND DIABETES

Possibly the most easily utilized treatment for adult onset diabetes is exercise. The physiology runs like this:

1. Muscles need energy to perform
2. The best energy source is glucose
3. Exercise increases the uptake of glucose by the muscle cell, which
4. Reduces blood glucose
5. Exercise also increases muscle mass, thus offering more glycogen storage, which
6. Further reduces blood glucose, and
7. A larger muscle mass creates a larger need for energy even when not exercising, thus
8. Helps to stabilize blood sugar

We have discussed the probability that the diabetic is often insulin-resistant, rather than insulin deficient. This explains why some diabetics have rather elevated insulin levels. Just as the fat cell becomes more insulin-receptive as it is reduced in size, so the muscle cell evidently becomes more insulin receptive when it is exercised. Thus the need for insulin can be dramatically decreased during exercise. If taking insulin, be careful in your beginning exercise routine and look for signs of hyperinsulinism.

A good exercise rule of thumb is to exercise a minimum of one-half hour, three times per week, at a rate adequate to raise your pulse rate at least to 120-140 beats per minute. Rapid walking is usually the very best exercise, vigorous dancing is also excellent. In fact, any exercise which uses the heavy muscles in the upper leg is good - according to Dr. Hans Kugler, such exercise is the best for burning off fat.

Let me give you some of the other benefits of excrcise:
1. Tones muscles
2. Improves circulation
3. Lowers cholesterol
4. Stimulates internal organs
5. Burns off fat
6. Eases stress
7. Chases depression
8. Improves sex
9. Promotes sleep
10. Helps you think better

I have personally found that the minitrampoline is the ideal exercise for me - convenient and efficient.

With so many benefits to your health and well being for so little expense, how can you afford not to stock up a few?

RECENT DEVELOPMENT

Another trace mineral recently determined to have a positive effect on diabetes is vanadium. Chromium increases cellular utilization of glucose by 16% whereas vanadium increases cellular utilization of glucose by 33%. Vanadium has shown such promise that investigators claim that vanadium supplementation will eliminate the need for insulin.

It has been known for some time that vanadium is an essential nutrient and that it regulates glucose, triglyceride and cholesterol metabolism. Early signs of vanadium deficiency include dry-brittle hair and elevated glucose, cholesterol and triglycerides; vanadium at 20 to 30 mg per day will bring these values into the normal range.

STRESS

There is a definite correlation between stress and diabetes, but it is not the major predisposing factor. Many potential or borderline diabetics will spill sugar in the urine during a period of high stress, but when the stress is relieved the sugar often recedes. It is a fact though, that most of these borderline diabetics who react to stress in this fashion will eventually become diagnosed, full-blown diabetics.

The most common stresses are traumatic injury, surgery, myocardial infarction, and pregnancy. Stress causes the release of certain hormones (cortisol, glucagon, catecholamines) which not only inhibit insulin secretion but increase the production of glucose by the liver from glycogen reserves. If there is no energy output to utilize the elevated blood glucose, the excess can easily be seen either in the urine or the blood. A fasting blood sugar level of over 120 mg/dl is indicative of the possibility of diabetes, the higher it goes, the more positive the diagnosis.

DRUG INDUCED DIABETES

Transient or temporary diabetes may be induced by any of a number of drugs. The corticosteroids are the most common (cortisone or any of its derivatives), birth control pills can be even more dangerous because of their daily use, and the diuretics are also a contributory to hyperglycemia, as is phenytoin sodium (dilantin). Alcohol, although not a prescription drug, also often produces high levels of blood/urine sugar.

Cortisone - This adrenal hormone is antagonistic to insulin, and its use, particularly to treat minor conditions such as acne, bursitis, and the like is seriously questioned by diabetic specialists who are aware of the ever increasing number of diabetics diagnosed each year.

Birth Control Pills - The carbohydrate intolerant female (and this includes the hypoglycemic) should have serious thoughts before she uses the birth control pill. The effect of oral contraceptives on the metabolism of carbohydrates and fats is profound. The manner in which the contraceptive pill works is to prevent ovulation by creating a state of pseudo pregnancy. It is the rule, rather than the exception, for this hormonal, contra-insulin internal environment to be maintained over an unnaturally long period of time while on the pill. Frankly, diabetic glucose tolerance tests are observed in 15 to 40 percent of the women on the pill. Lesser degrees of worsening of glucose tolerance are observed in up to 80 percent of these women. Insulin levels are actually increased in the presence of the pill; their diabetogenic action is a reflection of an induced increased resistance to the action of insulin. Although studies have shown that in 90 percent of a large test group there is improvement in carbohydrate tolerance after discontinuance of the pill, another study revealed that four out of five women who had a significant predisposition to diabetes continued to have abnormal glucose metabolism after they stopped using the pill. These are frightening statistics - frightening enough for me to advise any female reader who is predisposed to carbohydrate intolerance to find some other means of contraception.

Diuretics - These drugs do not affect the carbohydrate intolerant as significantly as the other drugs. Their prime function is to stimulate the excretion of water by the body. In so doing they can increase the concentration of glucose to a point where a borderline diabetic may become a clinical diabetic. Their indiscriminate use in weight loss programs where the individual already probably has a carbohydrate problem should be of concern.

THE GLUCOSE TOLERANCE TEST

The glucose tolerance test is considered by some physicians to be a simple and unequivocal test for diabetes. Many physicians now are seriously questioning such an attitude. The basic procedure involves drawing blood after fasting for at least 12 to 16 hours, then feeding a measured amount of glucose (standard is 75 gm for adults, 100 gm for pregnant females), and drawing blood at 30 minute to 1 hour intervals for from three to six hours. The resulting graph should be quite revealing as to how your body responds to a load of sugar. Because of recent research, an alternative test has been devised for those patients which are borderline or for which the physician wishes additional documentation.

Two-Hour Post-Prandial Test - The patient should not be on a low calorie diet, or a weight reducing diet, as this may cause his body to overreact to the sudden glucose load which any of these tests are based upon. For three days immediately preceeding the test the patient should use a special diet containing 250 grams of carbohydrate per day. Although this is high, it prevents carbohydrate shock from the test. On test day, the patient eats a breakfast of 6 ounces of orange juice, three hotcakes with syrup (made from sugar), and tea with two teaspoons of sugar. Two hours later, blood is drawn and if the plasma glucose level is above 250 mg/dl, the patient has diabetes.

Plasma Glucose Test - Simple plasma glucose tests are used by those physicians who are satisfied with fasting examination of the blood. The criteria is a fasting glucose level above 140 mg/dl.

DIETARY FIBER IN DIABETES

Recent times have made us aware of food factors that have been overlooked in our quest for a chemical answer to diabetes. Persons with diabetes mellitus may reap substantial benefits from increasing their intake of dietary fiber. The short term use of selected fibers lowers blood glucose values and insulin requirements, serum cholesterol and triglyceride values often also decline. The use of these foods high in fiber offers us two potential benefits. First, improved diabetic control should lessen the likelihood of the specific complications of diabetes, such as complications from infections, wounds, etc. Second, improved diabetic control coupled with lower serum cholesterol and triglyceride values should lessen the risk of arteriosclerotic, cardiovascular disease. Research evidence supports both of these suggested benefits.

In regions such as Japan, India, and the West Indies where the intake of carbohydrate dietary fiber is high, the specific complications of diabetes are less frequent than in Western countries, where the fiber intake is low. Heart attacks and diabetic gangrene among persons with diabetes are less common in India and Japan than in the United States. Thus, an increase in dietary fiber intake by persons with diabetes may improve diabetic control, and the risk for the small-blood-vessel complications specific for diabetes as well as for large-blood vessel disease may be decreased.

The evidence of the protective effect of dietary fiber is also encouraging. In countries where dietary fiber intake is high, the incidence of diabetes in general is much lower than in Western World nations where dietary fiber content in the diet is rather low.

The glucose lowering and insulin sparing effect that given quantities of fiber exhibit are probably due to the fact that fiber forms a "gel" in the intestinal tract and probably "holds" or "traps" for a period of time some of the sugars in the diet so that they are much more slowly absorbed through the gut. This "trickle" phenomenon was clearly demonstrated when a given amount of glucose was given to patients with and without a fiber substance. In every instance the fiber-glucose combination displayed lower blood glucose levels and lower insulin stimulation.

High Fiber Drink - A new high fiber protein powder which is to be drunk with each meal has been tested and is being used by a number of carbohydrate intolerants. The results for some have been nothing short of phenomenal -decrease or elimination of insulin, better healing, a feeling of vigor, etc. This is a positive step to insure the fiber content in a diet that is woefully short of the desired amounts. In order to produce the results that researchers found, it is necessary to have at least 35 to 45 grams of fiber in the diet per day.

HOW ABOUT VITAMINS AND MINERALS?

Although no simple answer exists for supplementation, the diabetic should pay careful attention to the Glucose Tolerance Factor mentioned before (chromium, niacin, glutamic acid), zinc, vitamin E, vitamin C, all the B complex and the rest of the essential minerals. Nutrition supplementation is a partnership arrangement with many different nutrients working in concert to achieve the proper end result. I must just mention here that in my research I found that a small percentage of individuals are diabetic not because of insulin deficiency, or insulin resistance, but because of poorly formed insulin. Many of these respond to an increase in the mineral zinc in their diet, since this mineral is essential in the proper formation of insulin.

The following formula would be recommended as a basic vitamin and mineral supplement for those afflicted with carbohydrate intolerance:

A Special Mega Potency Formulation

Vitamin A	25,000IU	Calcium	500 mg.
Vitamin D	1,000IU	Magnesium	250 mg.
Vitamin E	400IU	Phosphorus	100 mg.
Vitamin C	2,000 mg.	Potassium	99 mg.
Vitamin B_1	50 mg.	Iron (Ferrous Fumerate)	15 mg.
Vitamin B_2	50 mg.	Zinc (Chloride)	25 mg.
Vitamin B_6	100 mg.	Iodine (Kelp)	0.225 mg.
Vitamin B_{12}	500 mcg.	Copper (Gluconate)	1 mg.
Niacinamide	50 mg.	Chromium	200 mcg.
Pantothenic Acid	1,500 mg.	Manganese (Gluconate)	20 mg.
Folic Acid	400 mcg.	Bioflavonoids	100 mg.
Biotin	100 mcg.	Ribonucleic Acid	10 mg.
Choline	50 mg.	Betaine (HCl)	150 mg.
Inositol	100 mg.	Selenium	200 Mcg.
PABA	50 mg.	Glutamic Acid	200 mg.

Glandular Support - Carbohydrate intolerance, in whatever stage, is very hard on the cells of the entire body. One of the signs of a diabetic is a thickening of the "basement" membrane of the cell. This membrane is made up of collagen protein and a very tiny amount of glucose under normal conditions. In diabetes, the glucose content of the basement membrane begins to increase and as it does, it becomes spongy and thicker. Rather than becoming less permeable, it becomes more permeable, and precious nutrients leak out. In the case of tiny blood vessels, they tend to rupture very readily, leading to the eye problems so common in diabetics. In order to support the body in its restoration process, I have found it beneficial to add glandular extracts which facilitate the rebuilding of cells in specific glands and organs. Here are some sample formulae which might be used:

Formula For Female

Two tablets contain:

Ovarian Substance	60 mg.	Spleen Substance	60 mg.
Heart Substance	60 mg.	Adrenal Substance	60 mg.
Thymus Substance	60 mg.	Liver Substance	60 mg.
PABA	30 mg.	Whole Pituitary Sub.	10 mg.
RNA	40 mg.	Brain Substance	60 mg.
Kidney Substance	60 mg.	Pancreas Substance	60 mg.

Formula For Male

Two tablets contain:

Prostate Substance	60 mg.	Zinc	15 mg.
Brain Substance	60 mg.	Whole Pituitary Sub.	10 mg.
Pancreas Substance	60 mg.	Kidney Substance	60 mg.
PABA	30 mg.	Spleen Substance	60 mg.
Orchic Substance	60 mg.	Adrenal Substance	60 mg.
Heart Substance	60 mg.	Liver Substance	60 mg.
Thymus Substance	60 mg.	RNA	40 mg.

SUMMARY

Diabetes is a very controllable disease. In particular, adult onset diabetes, which is not caused by a loss of function of the beta cells of the pancreas, is very responsive to dictary control. The program is rather simple but very effective:

1. Reduce weight
2. Completely eliminate refined carbohydrates
3. Exercise regularly
4. Eliminate, if possible, the drugs which predispose one to diabetes - cortisone, birth control pills, diuretics, and alcohol
5. Increase the dietary fiber in your diet to a minimum of 35 to 45 grams per day
6. Use food supplements which contain the "glucose tolerance factor" and other essential nutrients for glucose metabolism
7. Glandular extracts can speed up your recovery

Your health is the greatest wealth you will ever own. Prompt attention to these matters could bring you a return beyond expectations.

Although many diabetics are quite familiar with normal blood sugar levels they often are unfamiliar with normals for the various fats in the blood - including cholesterol, triglycerides, and total lipids. These values are considered normal after an 8 to 12 hour fast. They often reflect, when increased, an inability of the body to properly metabolize glucose or fructose or both.

BLOOD VALUES

GLUCOSE	70-110 Mg.%
TOTAL LIPIDS	400-600 Mg.%
TRIGLYCERIDES	50-150 Mg.%
CHOLESTEROL	130-260 Mg.%

CALORIE CONSUMPTION RELATED TO ACTIVITY

Physical Exercise	Calories per Hour
Walking 2mph	200
3mph	270
4mph	350
Running	800-1000
Cycling 5mph	250
10mph	450
14mph	750
Horseback riding	
walk	150
trot	500
gallop	600
Dancing	200-400
Gymnastics	200-500
Golf	300
Tennis	400-500
Soccer	550
Sculling	
50 strokes per minute	420
97 strokes per minute	670
Rowing (peak effort)	1200
Swimming, breast and backstroke	300-650
crawl	700-900
Squash	600-700
Climbing	700-900
Skiing	600-700
Skating (fast)	300-700
Wrestling	900-1000

Domestic Occupations	
Sewing	10-30
Writing	20
Sitting at rest	15
Standing relaxed	20
Dressing and undressing	30-40
Ironing (with 5-lb. iron)	60
Dishwashing	60
Sweeping or dusting	80-130
Polishing	150-200

* These figures are based on the caloric consumption of a moderately obese person. A nonobese person would burn somewhat fewer calories per hour, a markedly obese one somewhat more.

HORMONAL INFLUENCES ON CARBOHYDRATE METABOLISM

Hormone	Effect on Insulin secretion	Effect on gluconeo-genesis in the liver	Effect on peripheral glucose utilization
Epinephrine	Decreases	Increases	Decreases
Cortisol	Increases	Increases	Decreases
Growth hormone	Increases	Increases	Decreases
Somatostatin	Decreases	No effect	No effect
Thyroid	No effect	No effect	Increases

UNDERSTANDING DIABETIC EMERGENCIES

People with poorly controlled diabetes are always at risk of two emergency situations. The first, *hypoglycemia,* or very low blood sugar, can occur in both type 1 (also called insulin-dependent or ketosis-prone) diabetes and type 2 (also called adult-onset, or ketosis-resistant) diabetes, but it is rare with type 2. The second, *diabetic ketoacidosis,* occurs only in type 1 diabetes. You and your family must be able to distinguish between these two emergencies. Since immediate treatment is always important and sometimes critical, protect yourself by learning to recognize early symptoms.

A summary of the following information on diabetic emergencies, for family use, particularly for the child onset, insulin dependent type which the text of this booklet did not cover, is provided.

HYPOGLYCEMIA
(Induced by Excess Insulin)

Causes: The amount of insulin you inject each day to control your diabetes has been determined from an estimate of your usual diet and level of physical activity. If you exercise less than usual, you may be getting more insulin than you need. This excess of insulin causes the blood sugar level to drop too low for your body to function normally. If you are taking an oral antidiabetes agent for type 2 diabetes, you may get hypoglycemia by missing meals, by unusual exercise, or by inadvertently taking too much of your oral medication.

How to recognize early clues.   Hypoglycemic reactions come on suddenly. Early signs differ from person to person, but any of these may occur:

☐ Mood change	☐ Hunger
☐ Trembling	☐ Sweating
☐ Pallor	☐ Light-headedness
☐ Pounding heartbeat	☐ Confusion and disorientation
☐ Drowsiness	☐ Inability to concentrate
☐ Inability to focus your eyes while reading or watching television.	

If hypoglycemia is allowed to progress, you may become unconscious.

What to do at the earliest sign. If you are exercising, *stop.* Immediately eat a simple, fast-acting sugar such as:

- [ ] A half cup of orange juice sweetened with 1 teaspoon of sugar, if handy.
- [ ] 6-7 Life Savers or other small candies.
- [ ] 2 teaspoons of sugar dissolved in a half cup of lukewarm water.
- [ ] Instant glucose.
- [ ] 1 tablespoon Karo or other corn syrup, honey, or maple syrup, alone or added to a half cup of orange juice.
- [ ] Any other available candy or sweet such as jam or jelly.

The most effective way to prevent the hypoglycemic emergency is to consume several small meals per day, particularly meals that contain significant protein and complex carbohydrates. Such a meal ½ hour before heavy exercise will often prevent any problem. The exercise induced hypoglycemia occurs because low levels of blood sugar brought about by insulin injection do not adequately supply the needs of the body rapidly enough. Increased activity increases the need for fuel which is manufactured by the liver and muscle cells and if this conversion process does not come about soon enough blood sugar levels can dip quite low.

What to do for a severe reaction. Your parents, teachers, family, and friends should be familiar with the symptoms of a hypoglycemia reaction and should know what to do if it becomes severe. The first step is to give sugar. In case you are unable to swallow, they should know how to give you an injection of glucagon. Instructions for your family on injecting glucagon follow.

DIABETIC KETOACIDOSIS AND COMA

Causes: Diabetic ketoacidosis may result from unusual and/or prolonged stress to your body caused by illness, an accident, surgery, or, perhaps, severe emotional stress.

The immediate effect of this stress is a greatly increased blood sugar level. Also, excessive amounts of stress hormones are excreted; they further increase the blood sugar level by lowering the insulin supply. Since your insulin supply is inadequate to handle this high level of blood sugar, your body gets the heat and energy it needs by "burning" large amounts of fats in a process called fat metabolism. Products of fat metabolism—ketones—ordinarily are well utilized by the body, but under these circumstances, so many ketones are produced that they back up into the blood. Some of these ketones are acid; they acidify the blood, leading to ketoacidosis.

How to recognize early clues: Ketoacidosis develops slowly over 8-24 hours. At first, there may be no symptoms. To detect it as early as possible, conscientiously test your urine as often as your doctor recommends—at least every day without fail. The first warning signs are tests showing large amounts of sugar—1-2 percent—in your urine, accompanied by a positive test for urinary ketones. At this point, call you doctor immediately.

During the early stages of ketoacidosis, you may also experience excessive thirst, excessive urination, and often nausea, vomiting, stomach pains, and rapid breathing. Later, you may feel drowsy, and your breath will have a fruity odor. You are sick and your body is telling you so.

Remember that an infection, fever, or intestinal upset increases your body's need for insulin and can cause ketoacidosis to develop quickly. If you become ill, be sure to continue testing your urine and increase your insulin dosage if test results are high. Your doctor has already given you instructions for adjusting your insulin dosage if you have several successive positive urine tests. Call him if you are vomiting, if signs of ketoacidosis accompany your illness, of if you have trouble adjusting your insulin dosage. If you become stuporous or unconscious, you should be taken to the hospital immediately.

EMERGENCY TREATMENT

Hypoglycemia	Ketoacidosis
CAUSES	
Too much insulin or oral hypoglycemic drug	Not enough insulin
Not enough food because of skimpy, skipped, or delayed meals	
More exercise than usual	Possibly, severe emotional stress
ONSET	
Sudden	Gradual
SIGNS	
No sugar in urine	Sugar and ketones in urine
Mood change	Increased thirst and urination
Confusion and disorientation	Weakness, drowsiness
Hunger	Loss of appetite
Pounding heartbeat	Nausea, vomiting
Pallor	Stomach pain
Light-headedness	Sweet-smelling breath
Blurry vision	Rapid breathing
Sweating	Stupor
Trembling	Unconsciousness
Drowsiness	
TREATMENT	
See that the patient consumes sugar.*	Call a doctor
If he is unable to swallow, give glucagon.	If no doctor is available, take patient to the hospital.
If patient is not alert and able to take food within 25 minutes after the glucagon injection, take him to the hospital.	
POSTEMERGENCY CARE	
Discuss insulin or oral hypoglycemic dosage with doctor.	

*Such as 2 teaspoons of sugar dissolved in a half cup of lukewarm water.

HOW TO ADMINISTER GLUCAGON

Glucagon is a hormone that quickly raises the blood sugar. If a patient's hypoglycemic reaction is so severe that he cannot swallow, you may have to give him a glucagon injection. Even though this is a rare emergency, you should have glucagon available and know how to administer it.

1. You will need:

> Glucagon package (store in a cool place)*
> Disposable syringe and needle (you may use an insulin syringe and needle)
> Alcohol Sponge packets
> Adhesive bandage
> Sugar packets
> Paper cup

* Be sure to keep track of the expiration date of your glucagon supply. The date is printed clearly on the back of the carton. As that date approaches, discard your old bottle of glucagon and replace it with a new one.

2. *In the glucagon package* you will find two numbered bottles. One bottle (bottle number 1) contains diluting fluid; the other (bottle number 2) contains either a tablet of glucagon or glucagon powder.

3. *Clean the rubber caps* of the bottles with an alcohol sponge. Then insert the sterile needle through the rubber cap of bottle number 1 and pull the plunger to withdraw all the diluting fluid.

4. *Insert the needle* into the rubber cup of bottle number 2 and inject the fluid into the bottle with the tablet or powder. Leave syringe in the bottle (a).

5. *Shake the bottle* for a few seconds to dissolve the tablet or powder. Then invert the bottle and draw all of the dissolved glucagon into the syringe by pulling back on the plunger (b).

6. *With the second alcohol sponge,* cleanse an area on the front of the patient's thigh about midway between the hip and the knee.

7. *Hold the barrel of the syringe* and push the needle *quickly* through the cleansed area of skin at about a 45-degree angle. Push the needle in all the way to the hub.

8. *Push steadily down on the plunger while holding the syringe barrel steady. Inject the entire contents of the syringe.*

9. *Pull the needle quickly* from the leg. If bleeding occurs, cover the puncture site with an adhesive bandage.

10. *The patient should recover within about 15 minutes* after you inject the glucagon. As soon as he can swallow, give him a teaspoon or packet of sugar dissolved in a half glass of lukewarm water or some other easily swallowed food containing sugar. Repeat this 10-15 minutes later. *This step is very important.* If he does not eat or drink something—even though he has recovered from the reaction—he's likely to have another reaction. If he is not alert and able to eat 25 minutes after the glucagon injection, take him to the hospital. Be sure that you report any nausea or vomiting.

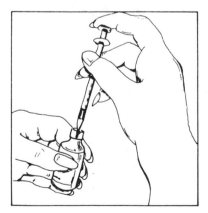 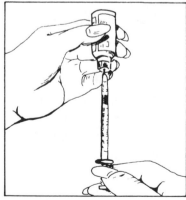

(NON-DIABETIC)

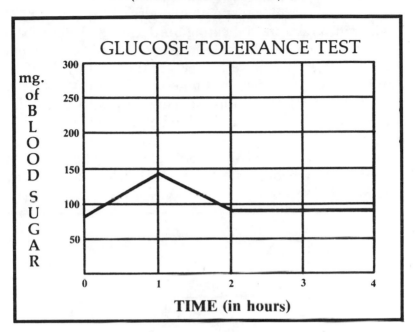

(DIABETIC)

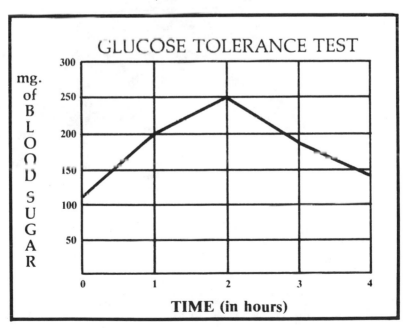

Oral glucose tolerance test levels
diagnostic of diabetes.

The wide gray zone indicating borderline diabetes is based on the range of plasma glucose values obtained from several sources. The lowest levels are those set by the U.S. Public Health Service; the highest, those of Marvin D. Siperstein, M.D., diabetologist, University of California, San Francisco. Obtain whole blood glucose values by subtracting 15 percent.

Levels in this table are not applicable during pregnancy; see table on the opposite page for levels diagnostic of gestational diabetes.

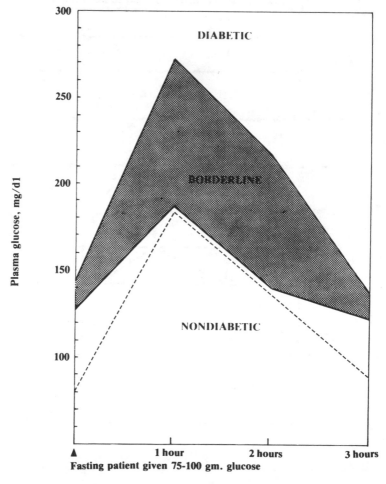

* The dotted line is the authors opinion of normal.

Oral glucose tolerance test levels
diagnostic of gestational diabetes.

The 100 gm glucose loading dose is utilized for pregnant patients. The three-hour value does not drop to fasting levels, as in nonpregnant patients.

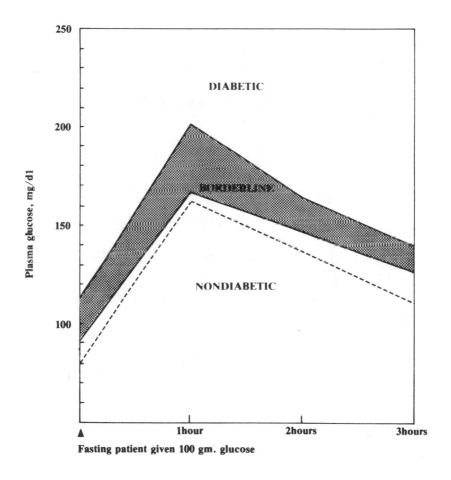

* Dotted lines indicate authors concept of normal.

BIBLIOGRAPHY

1. Diabetes - New Look At An Old Problem, Lowenstein & Preger, Harper & Row.

2. Human Nutrition, Benjamin T. Burton, McGraw-Hill.

3. Nutrition and Diabetes Mellitus, Anderson & Kaufman, School of Public Health, University of North Carolina.

4. Sugar: "Sweet and Dangerous," Linus Pauling, Executive Health, Vol. IX, No. 1.

5. Diabetes: Deeper Insight, Surer Control, Drs. Bid, Clark, Ensinck, McLain, Olson, Wishner, Patient Care, The Practical Journal For Primary Physicians, Vol. 14, No.5.

6. Diabetes Mellitus, Seventh Edition, Lilly Research Laboratories.

7. Diabetes, The Medical Clinics of North America, White, Volume 49, No. 4, W.B. Saunders Company

8. Diabetes, The New Approach, Brothers, Grosset & Dunlap.

9. Medical Aspects of Dietary Fiber, Spiller & Kay, Plenum Medical Book Company.

10. The Saccharine Disease, Cleave, John Wright and Sons, Ltd.

11. Influence of Nutritional Factors on Prevalence of Diabetes, West & Kalbfleisch, Diabetes 20:99-108, 1971.

12. Nutrition in the Prevention and Treatment of Disease.

EMBRACING WHOLISTIC HEALTH

By Kurt W. Donsbach, D.C., N.D., Ph.D.

CLARIFYING THE
BODY-MIND-SPIRIT
CONNECTION
in
CANCER • ARTHRITIS • CANDIDIASIS
HEART DISEASE • MULTIPLE SCLEROSIS

Explicit treatment protocols from the world famous natural healing institutions - Hospital Santa Monica, Hospital St. Augustine and Institut Santa Monica

You can order this 300 page profusely illustrated manual by checking with your local health food store or calling 1-800-423-7662. Total Cost: $17.95. Dr. Donsbach feels this is his best work yet. You should have this book on your shelf to help you answer health questions that may come up. It is the best review of the application and merits of wholistic health philosophy available today.